Aromatherapy
OILS

Written and designed by Ark Creative

KUDOS

Published by Kudos, an imprint of Top That! Publishing plc.
Copyright © 2004 Top That! Publishing plc,
Tide Mill Way, Woodbridge, Suffolk, IPI2 IAP. www.kudosbooks.com

Kudos is a Trademark of Top That! Publishing plc.

2

Contents

What are Aromatherapy Oils?	4	Evening Primrose	36
Aromatics through the Ages	6	Grapeseed	38
In the Mood	8	Jojoba	40
Rest and Relaxation	10	Peach Kernel	42
Sensual Calm	12	Sweet Almond	44
Room Perfume	14	Infused Oils	46
Peaches and Cream	16	Top 20 Essential Oils	48
Heady Scents	18	Camomile	50
Bed of Roses	20	Cedarwood Atlas	52
Music to your Senses	22	Clary Sage	54
Harmonising starts Here	24	Cypress and Eucalyptus	56
A Symphony of Scents	26	Frankincense	58
Carrier Oils	28	Geranium	60
Apricot Kernel	30	Grapefruit	62
Avocado	32	Lavender	64
Borage	34	Lemon	66

Lime	68	Ginger	100
Mandarin	70	Jasmine and Juniper	102
Neroli	72	Lemon grass	104
Orange	74	Marjoram	106
Peppermint	76	Myrrh	108
Rose Otto	78	Niaouli and Palmarosa	110
Rosemary	80	Patchouli	112
Sandalwood	82	Petitgrain	114
Tea Tree	84	Rosewood	116
Ylang Ylang	86	Spearmint	118
Diffuse your Dreams	88	Tangerine	120
Basil	90	Thyme	122
Bay	92	Vetiver	124
Black Pepper and Citronella	94	Dos and Don'ts	126
Clove Bud	96	Caring for your Oils	128
Fennel	98		

Aromatherapy oils, also known as 'essential' or 'volatile' oils, are the highly fragrant liquid components of aromatic plants, trees and grasses. They can be found in different parts of the plant including the petals (rose), bark (cinnamon), resin (frankincense) and leaves (eucalyptus).

The term 'aromatherapy' dates back to the 1920s when French cosmetic chemist René-Maurice Gattefossé discovered the healing properties of essential oils.

He suffered severe burns to his hand in a laboratory explosion and treated the wound with undiluted lavender essence. It healed without a scar. Essential oils were found to contain powerful antiseptic and pain-killing properties.

At that time, Italian doctors, Gatti and Cajola, demonstrated the therapeutic effects of smelling essential oils. The holistic use of essential oils was further developed in the 1950s when Austrian-born Marguerite Maury introduced the idea of combining them with massage.

The true founders of aromatherapy are thought to be the ancient Egyptians. They extracted aromatic oils from exotic flowers by squeezing the oil from the petals. The preservative powers of the oils made them an essential part of the embalming process, and they were also blended into perfumes and used as incense.

The Greeks advocated the wearing of fragrant garlands and of taking daily aromatic baths, and soon the Romans too were extolling the virtues of healing balms and aromatherapy massage.

Persian physician Avicenna
believed that plant essences
strengthened body and spirit,
and the Persians developed a
passion for the perfume derived
from the essential oil of
red roses.

In ancient China, Chinese
alchemists believed that plant
extracts contained magical forces
to help them develop the elixir
of life!

Knowing a little about the origins of essential oils, you'll be keen to practise the ancient art of aromatherapy for yourself. It's the perfect way to achieve peace of mind – think of it as nature's antidote to stress!

Create your own calming space by using incense sticks or cones to scent your room. Candles complement the theme – especially when they are scented. Specially designed holders should be used for both candles and incense.

Why not make your own aromatic candle? It's best to buy a chunky beeswax candle to give you the added benefit of honeyed scent! Light it and wait for the wax around the wick to melt. Then blow it out and carefully add a few drops of the essential oil to the molten wax BEFORE relighting.

Warning

Essential oils are highly flammable so NEVER add the oil while the candle is burning.

Rest and

Relaxation

At the end of a long day, prepare to kick off your shoes and slide into a warm fragrant bath. This is an excellent way to indulge in essential oils as you'll absorb the oils through your nose and skin.

- ✿ Blend 600 ml of carrier oil with 20 drops of your favourite smelling essential oil
- ✿ Store in an amber or cobalt glass bottle
- ✿ Run the bath first (otherwise the vapour will evaporate before you get in)
- ✿ Sprinkle 6 drops of oil on to the water's surface and agitate to disperse well
- ✿ Immerse yourself in heavenly scent!

Warning

Essential oils enter the bloodstream through the skin. NEVER apply them directly to your skin as they can be extremely potent. Dilute in a carrier oil and ALWAYS do a patch test first.

Patch test:

- Mix one drop of the essential oil into a teaspoon of carrier oil
- Rub a little of the mixture on the inside of your wrist
- Leave uncovered and unwashed for 24 hours
- If you suffer no redness or itching the oil is safe to use in a diluted form

Treat your partner to an aromatherapy massage – it will arouse the most primitive senses of smell and touch. Diluted in a carrier oil, then massaged into the skin, essential oils are sure to give the desired spine-tingling effect.

Make your own massage oil by mixing 8–10 drops of skin-friendly essential oil to 30 ml of carrier oil. Try blending 2 drops of rose otto with 5 drops of sandalwood for a truly sensuous massage.

Tip!

For a superior quality massage, seek 'unrefined' carrier oils that still contain their natural vitamins and skin enriching minerals.

Room

Perfume

Oil burners are a wonderful way to bring harmony into your home.

- ☸ Simply pour some water into the reservoir (this will prevent the oil from heating too quickly)
- ☸ Add some drops of your preferred essential oil
- ☸ Light a candle and place underneath to heat the reservoir
- ☸ As the water heats, the oil will gently warm through and your room will be redolent with gorgeous scent!

Warning

The fragranced oils included with this set are not essential oils, they have been specially designed and are for use ONLY with the oil burner. They are NOT for use on the skin.

After a bath or shower, your skin is warm and receptive and essential oils will be absorbed quickly. Make the most of it by treating yourself to a homemade massage oil that matches your skin type.

Warning

Remember the potency of these essential oils – patch test your skin before applying and NEVER apply undiluted.

Normal Skin

Mix 25 ml jojoba oil with 3 drops of lavender and 2 drops of neroli.

Dry Skin

Mix 25 ml peach nut oil with 1 drop of camomile, 4 drops of lavender, and 10 ml of avocado.

Sensitive Skin

Mix 30 ml almond oil with 1 drop of camomile.

Oily Skin

Mix 25 ml jojoba oil with 3 drops of cedarwood and 2 drops of frankincense.

NOTE
5 ml is equal to 1 teaspoon.
Adjust accordingly.

Heady

Many carrier oils make wonderful conditioning treatments for your hair. Choose from jojoba, peach kernel and extra virgin olive oil to give your hair a lustrous shine.

Select your hair type from the list opposite and see which essential oils are best suited to you.

Tip!

Add 2 drops of rosemary or sandalwood to the bristles of your hairbrush and brush through your hair. Heady scents indeed!

Normal Hair
Geranium, lavender, mandarin, neroli, petitgrain and rose otto

Dry Hair
Camomile, sandalwood, jojoba and ylang ylang

Fine Hair
Patchouli and rosemary

Greasy Hair
Eucalyptus, grapefruit, lemon, tea tree and cypress

The seductive power

of scent and the way in which it lifts our spirits is rooted deep within us – whether it's the smell of newly mown grass, the mouth-watering smell of baking in the kitchen, or the crisp clean fragrance of fresh laundry.

Bring a woody fragrance to your laundry by adding some drops of frankincense or sandalwood to the distilled water in your steam iron.

For restful sleep and sweet dreams mix 15 drops of rose otto or lavender oil to 125 ml of water and spray over your bed linen.

Keep drawers fresh by lining them with wallpaper that has first been cut to size and sprayed with a strong aromatic concentrate of your chosen essential oil (40 drops to 50 ml of water).

Tip!

If you have an open fire perfume the room by burning aromatic plants such as lavender flowers and rosemary twigs.

Music to your senses

Perfume notes were the creation of nineteenth century French perfumer Charles Piesse. He categorised the aroma of essential oils to relate to a scale of top, middle and base notes, like those of a musical stave.

The perfume industry still uses these three categories today – a good blend of perfume is a well-balanced combination of top, middle and base notes.

Tip!

Base notes 'fix' the fragrance and make it last longer.

In aromatherapy, the top (head) notes are the most volatile essential oils because they are fast-acting and evaporate quickly. Middle (heart) notes are therapeutic and balancing, and base (bottom) notes are the least volatile oils that have a long-lasting effect.

Stimulating your senses, the top note is what you smell first. This fades away leaving you with the heart note and when this too fades, you can still smell the bottom note which lingers long after the other two have gone.

Have a go at composing your own perfumes by experimenting with different blends of aromatic notes. Some scents stand out as popular solo artists on their own and you may not want to blend these with anything at all. Rose otto, ylang ylang, jasmine and patchouli are the most common of these.

With so many oils to choose from, it's helpful to know that essences can be categorised into their own musical 'family' and that as a rule, aromatic notes from the same family harmonise well together.

Tip!

The Victorian era popularised the use of essential oils as a tonic to lift the spirits. You too can benefit by adapting their recipe for smelling salts – just mix a few drops of your favourite scented oil with some rock salt. Orange and patchouli is the perfect pick-me-up!

Start creating your symphony by selecting 2–4 drops of essential oils from the same family, then dilute them in 10 ml of carrier oil.

THE AROMATIC FAMILY

CITRUS	FLORAL	HERBACEOUS	* CAMPHORACEOUS
grapefruit	geranium	camomile	eucalyptus
lemon	camomile	lavender	rosemary
lime	rose otto	peppermint	peppermint
mandarin	lavender	rosemary	tea tree
orange	ylang ylang	marjoram	lavender
	neroli	clary sage	

Scents

SPICY	RESINOUS	WOODY	EARTHY
black pepper	frankincense	cedarwood	patchouli
ginger	myrrh	sandalwood	vetiver
		juniper	
		cypress	

* Camphoraceous aromatics are medicinal and contain counterirritant, healing and antiseptic properties. They may also be used in the treatment of colds.

Carrier oils (sometimes called vegetable, base, or fixed oils) are derived from the fatty portions of seeds, nuts, vegetables and plants. These are the base oils used to dilute essential oils before applying them to the skin, so called because they 'carry' the essential oil onto your skin.

Carrier oils do not evaporate when heated, neither do they impart their aroma as strongly as essential oils. For this reason always try to obtain 'cold pressed' or 'extra virgin' carrier oils as these will contain the most therapeutic properties.

All carrier oils make excellent choices for massage as they are rich in nutrients and moisturising properties.

Tip!

Purchase carrier oils in small quantities as their shelf life is only three months.

Apricot Kernel

Plant: Apricot Kernel

Botanical name: Prunus armeniaca

Origins: Extracted from the seed kernel of the fruit.

Aroma: Faint smell of marzipan.

Properties: Light textured, easily absorbed, contains vitamins A and C.

Uses: A special oil used mainly in beauty care, and an excellent base for a face or body massage.

Plant: Avocado

Botanical name: Persea americana

Origins: Best quality is cold pressed from the flesh of the fruit.

Aroma: Faintly nutty.

Properties: Highly penetrative, rich in essential fatty acids, betacarotene and vitamin E.

Uses: A special oil used mainly in beauty care – excellent for dry, ageing skin, or skin dehydrated by too much sunbathing!

Borage

Plant: Borage

Botanical name: Borago officinalis

Origins: Warm pressed or solvent extracted from the tiny seeds of the beautiful blue starflower plant – is often labelled 'Starflower' for this reason.

Aroma: Light and sweet.

Properties: Rich source of essential fatty acids.

Uses: A special oil used mainly in beauty care. The best way to enhance your skin is to take 'Starflower' capsules as a nutritional supplement.

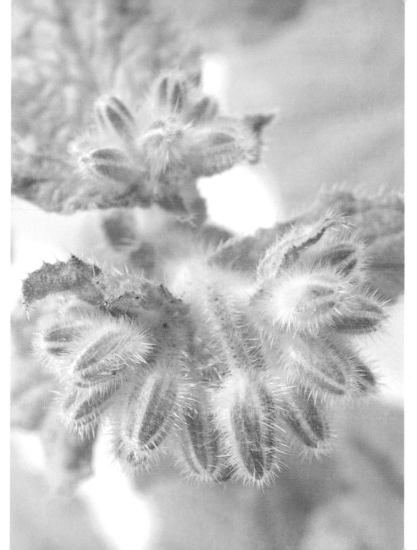

Plant: Evening Primrose

Botanical name: Oenothera biennis

Origins: Extracted from the tiny seeds of the bright yellow flowers which bloom only at night.

Aroma: Faint and musty.

Properties: Contains vitamins, minerals and essential fatty acids.

Uses: A nutritional supplement to treat premenstrual syndrome, period pains, arthritis and rheumatism. It is also excellent as a moisturising beauty treatment.

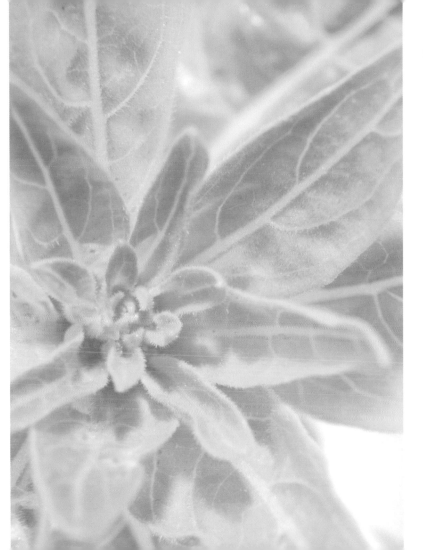

Plant: Grapeseed

Botanical name: Vitis vinifera

Origins: Heat extracted from the seeds of the fruit.

Aroma: Hardly any.

Properties: Heat extraction destroys the nutrients.

Uses: This is a popular massage oil.

Plant: Jojoba

Botanical name: Simmondsia chinensis

Origins: Liquid wax extracted from the beans of the plant.

Aroma: Hardly any.

Properties: Highly penetrative, also has some anti-inflammatory properties.

Uses: A special oil used mainly in beauty care. It is an excellent moisturiser for all skin types, and makes a good conditioning treatment for dry hair.

Peach Kernel

Plant: Peach Kernel

Botanical name: Prunus persica

Origins: Best quality is cold pressed from the kernels of the fruit.

Aroma: Delicate peachy aroma.

Properties: Fine textured so easily absorbed into the skin.

Uses: A special oil used mainly in beauty care, peach kernel oil is ideal for facial massage since it's kind to the skin. It will also add shine to hair.

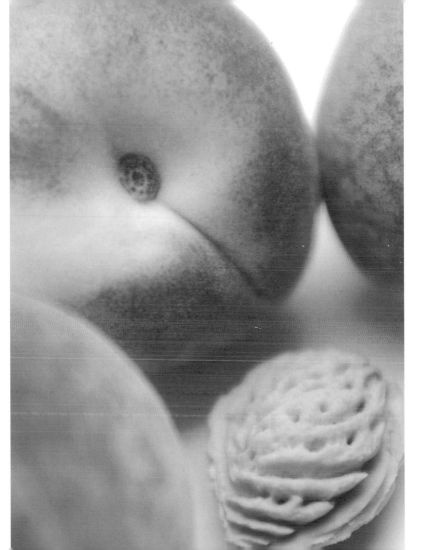

Plant: Sweet Almond

Botanical name: Prunus dulcis

Origins: Extracted from the kernels of the sweet almond tree.

Aroma: Faint nutty scent.

Properties: Contains vitamins D and E, also has some anti-inflammatory properties.

Uses: It is excellent for treating psoriasis, eczema and dermatitis – or to relieve sunburn.

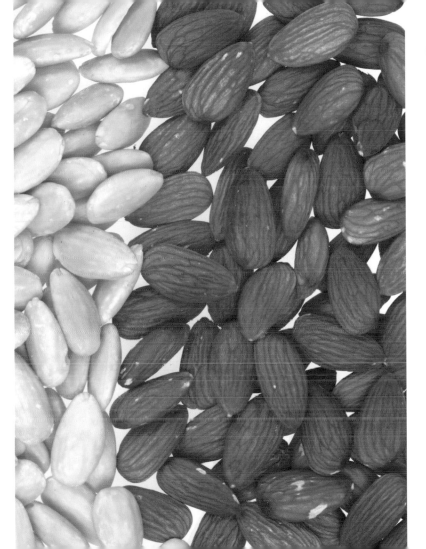

Infused

oils

Infused oils, sometimes called 'macerated' oils, are commercially made when the amount of essential oil in the plant is very small and therefore expensive to extract. Fresh plant matter is soaked or 'macerated' in a high quality carrier oil so that the essential oils are dissolved and impart their fragrance.

Plant: Hypericum (or St John's Wort)

Botanical name: Hypericum perforatum

Part used: Leaves and flowers.

Properties: Anti-inflammatory, anti-rheumatic.

Uses: It will ease rheumatism, sciatica, sunburn and bruises.

Plant: Calendula (or marigold)

Botanical name: Calendula officinalis

Part used: Flowers

Properties: Anti-inflammatory, antifungal.

Uses: This is excellent for treating eczema and nappy rash and soothes sore, inflamed and itchy skin.

Now you know what constitutes a carrier oil and what is meant by an infused oil, you're ready to try your hand at blending and experimenting with some aromatic oils of your choice! Take your pick from the 'Top 20' we've selected for you. Don't forget to try composing some subtle harmonies of your own by blending some top, middle and base notes together to compose a fragrant signature.

Plant: Camomile

Botanical name: Anthemis nobilis

Origins: Extracted from the flower heads.

Aroma: Sweet and fruity.

Properties: Anti-inflammatory and antiseptic.

Uses: A good treatment for premenstrual syndrome, insect bites, stings, insomnia and eczema.

Suggested Blends: Lavender, geranium, jasmine, rose otto and neroli.

Perfume Note: Middle

> **WARNING!**
> Do NOT use if you are pregnant.

Plant: Cedarwood Atlas

Botanical name: Anthemis nobilis

Origins: Distilled from the wood shavings and sawdust.

Aroma: Sweet and woody.

Properties: Antiseptic, astringent and sedative.

Uses: A good treatment for cystitis, fungal infections, dandruff, insect bites and stings.

Suggested Blends: Frankincense, ylang ylang, vetiver, juniper and rosemary.

Perfume Note: Base

Clary Sage

Plant: Clary Sage

Botanical name: Salvia sclarea

Origins: Distilled from the leaves and flower tops.

Aroma: Fruity and flowery.

Properties: Antidepressant, sedative and anti-inflammatory.

Uses: Clary sage can reduce high blood pressure, and ease depression, nervous tension and stress.

Suggested Blends: Lavender, tea tree and sandalwood.

Perfume Note: Middle

Plant: Cypress

Botanical name: Cupressus sempervirens

Origins: Distilled from the needles and twigs of young branches.

Aroma: Soft, piney and woody.

Properties: Astringent, antiseptic and antispasmodic.

Uses: This is valuable for treating varicose veins, menstruation and menopausal problems.

Suggested Blends: Clary sage, frankincense, juniper and lemon grass.

Perfume Note: Middle

Plant: Eucalyptus

Botanical name: Eucalyptus globulus

Origins: Distilled from the leaves and young twigs.

Aroma: Strong camphoraceous (medicinal) smell.

Properties: Antiseptic, anti rheumatic and analgesic.

Uses: Nature's first aid treatment for cuts, bruises and blisters. It is also excellent for coughs, colds, throat infections and congestion.

Suggested Blends: Lavender, tea tree, sandalwood and rosemary.

Perfume Note: Top

WARNING! NEVER take orally as it is very toxic.

Plant: Frankincense

Botanical name: Boswellia carterii

Origins: Extracted from the gum resin which collects when incisions are made into the bark.

Aroma: Piney, with a hint of camphor.

Properties: Astringent, antiseptic and sedative.

Uses: A good treatment for abscesses, ulcers, asthma and bronchitis.

Suggested Blends: Grapefruit, patchouli, rose otto and juniper.

Perfume Note: Base

Geranium

Plant: Geranium

Botanical name: Pelargonium odoratissimum

Origins: Distilled from the leaves, stalks and flowers

Aroma: Rose-scented, sweet and heavy.

Properties: Analgesic, antiseptic and astringent.

Uses: An excellent treatment for premenstrual syndrome, stress, cuts and skin problems.

Suggested Blends: Grapefruit, orange, lavender and neroli.

Perfume Note: Middle

Plant: Grapefruit

Botanical name: Citrus paradisi odoratissimum

Origins: Extracted from the fresh fruit peel.

Aroma: Clean, sharp citrus tang.

Properties: Digestive, antiseptic and astringent.

Uses: A good treatment for oily skin, acne and cellulite.

Suggested Blends: Orange, tangerine, peppermint and neroli.

Perfume Note: Top

Plant: Lavender

Botanical name: Lavandula augustifolia

Origins: Distilled from the flowering shrub tips.

Aroma: Sweet, flowery and herbaceous.

Properties: Analgesic, sedative and antiseptic.

Uses: Nature's first aid treatment for burns because it accelerates cell growth and repair. It has remarkable healing properties and can be used to alleviate high blood pressure and stress.

Suggested Blends: Rose otto, geranium, patchouli, rosemary and frankincense.

Perfume Note: Top/Middle

Lemon

number 10

Plant: Lemon

Botanical name: Citrus limon

Origins: Extracted from the peel of the fruit.

Aroma: Fresh and sharp.

Properties: Insecticidal, astringent and anti-rheumatic.

Uses: Excellent for oily skin, brittle nails, arthritis and rheumatism.

Suggested Blends: Chamomile, tangerine, juniper, myrrh and petitgrain.

Perfume Note: Top

CAUTION! Lemon oil only keeps for about six months.

Plant: Lime

Botanical name: Citrus aurantifolia

Origins: Extracted from the peel of the fruit.

Aroma: Bright, fresh and citrus.

Properties: Antiseptic and restorative.

Uses: To treat colds, depression and stress.

Suggested Blends:
Lavender, rosemary, grapefruit and orange.

Perfume Note: Top

CAUTION!
Lime oil only keeps for about six months.

Plant: Mandarin

Botanical name: Citrus nobilis

Origins: Extracted from the peel of the fruit.

Aroma: Sweet and citrus.

Properties: Digestive, laxative, and sedative.

Uses: This is good for children's problems such as colic, hiccups and coughs. It will also help to prevent stretch marks during pregnancy.

Suggested Blends: Lemon grass, rose otto, lemon and grapefruit.

Perfume Note: Top

Neroli

Plant: Neroli

Botanical name: Citrus aurantium

Origins: Distilled from the blossom of the orange tree.

Aroma: Sweet and floral.

Properties: Antidepressant and antiseptic. It's also reputed to be an aphrodisiac!

Uses: An excellent remedy for stress, skin care and heart palpitations.

Suggested Blends: Ginger, jasmine, lavender and orange.

Perfume Note: Middle

number 14

Plant: Orange

Botanical name: Citrus sinensis

Origins: Extracted from the peel of the fruit.

Aroma: Deliciously orangy.

Properties: Antidepressant and a tonic.

Uses: Will balance the digestive system and helps to lower blood pressure.

Suggested Blends: Clary sage, lavender and ginger.

Perfume Note: Top

CAUTION!
Orange oil only keeps for about six months.

Peppermint

> **WARNING!**
> Do NOT use
> if you are
> pregnant.

Plant: Peppermint

Botanical name: Mentha piperita

Origins: Distilled from the flower tops.

Aroma: Mint-scented and fresh.

Properties: Anti-inflammatory, antiseptic, and digestive.

Uses: It's excellent for indigestion, nausea, diarrhoea, colitis and sinus congestion. Will also make a good mosquito repellent.

Suggested Blends: Rosemary, lavender, eucalyptus and lemon.

Perfume Note: Top

Plant: Rose Otto

Botanical name: Rosa damascena

Origins: Distilled from the fresh rose petals.

Aroma: Sweet, with a hint of vanilla.

Properties: Sedative, antidepressant and a tonic.

Uses: Rose-water is a popular skin tonic. It is also used to combat menstrual disorders and stress.

Suggested Blends: Ylang ylang, geranium, patchouli, camomile, and frankincense.

Perfume Note: Middle to top

Rosemary

number 17

WARNING!
Do NOT use
if you are
either
pregnant or
epileptic.

Plant: Rosemary

Botanical name:
Rosmarinus officinalis

Origins: Steam distilled from the flowering tops of the plant.

Aroma: Camphoraceous and balsamic.

Properties: Anti-rheumatic and fungicidal.

Uses: Helps prevent dandruff and adds lustre to your hair. Will also ease muscular pain.

Suggested Blends: Tea tree, eucalyptus, geranium and peppermint.

Perfume Note: Middle

Sandalwood

Plant: Sandalwood

Botanical name: Santalum album

Origins: Distilled from the tree.

Aroma: Soft, sweet and woody.

Properties: Antiseptic, anti-inflammatory and antidepressant.

Uses: Used to treat stress, nausea, colic, and catarrh. It is invaluable for dry or inflamed skin.

Suggested Blends: Patchouli, cedarwood, rose otto, bay and vetiver.

Perfume Note: Base

Tea Tree

Plant: Tea Tree

Botanical name: Melaleuca alternifolia

Origins: Distilled from the leaves and twigs of the tree.

Aroma: Strongly medicinal.

Properties: Antibiotic, antiseptic and fungicidal.

Uses: Nature's first aid for fungal infections such as thrush and athlete's foot. An excellent treatment for mouth ulcers, cold sores, insect bites and stings.

Suggested Blends: Lavender, rosemary, spearmint and geranium.

Perfume Note: Middle

Plant: Ylang Ylang

Botanical name: Cananga odorata

Origins: Steam distilled from the freshly picked flowers.

Aroma: A heady floral mix of almonds and jasmine.

Properties: Sedative, tonic and antiseptic.

Uses: Used to treat stress, premenstrual syndrome, and nervous tension. A reputed aphrodisiac!

Suggested Blends: Black pepper, lemon, mandarin, grapefruit, and vetiver.

Perfume Note: Base

Diffuse your Dreams

Achieving dreamy room fragrances is easy! Your bedroom will be seductively transformed with a hint of any of the following essential oils, which can all be used with a lamp ring.

A lamp ring is a small, circular ring (metal or ceramic) that sits on top of an upward pointing light bulb. A few drops of your preferred aromatic oil can be dropped on to the ring so that the scent evaporates into the room as it heats up.

You could also try using an electric diffuser. This contains an electric heating element to warm a container for your oils, or by passing air from a fan

through an absorbent pad on to
which you have dropped
some oil.

Alternatively, make your own
personal diffuser.
Drop some oil on to a pad of
cotton wool and place inside a
small tin with holes in the lid.
Position on a radiator to
perfume the room.

Tip!

Lamp rings are NOT
recommended for light bulbs
stronger than 60 watts.

Basil

Plant: Basil

Botanical name: Ocimum basilicum

Origins: Steam distilled from the flower tops and leaves.

Aroma: Sweet and herb-scented.

Properties: Antiseptic, restorative and antidepressant.

Uses: This is good for respiratory problems, anxiety, depression, insect bites and coughs.

Suggested Blends: Clary sage, frankincense, geranium and neroli.

Perfume Note: Top

WARNING!
Do NOT use
if you are
pregnant.

Plant: Bay

Botanical name: Laurus nobilis

Origins: Extracted from the leaves.

Aroma: Spicy and medicinal smelling.

Properties: Restorative and a tonic.

Uses: This is a good treatment for aching muscles, coughs, colds and rheumatism.

Suggested Blends: Lavender, tea tree and frankincense.

Perfume Note: Middle

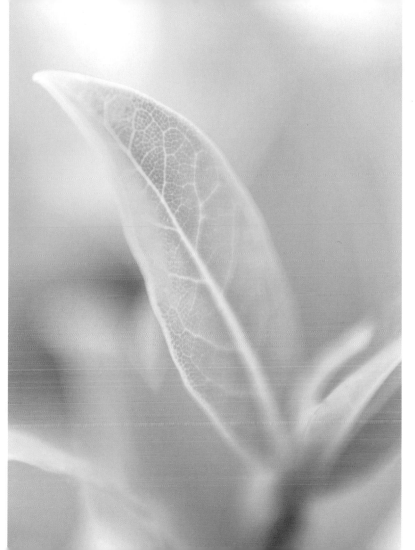

Black Pepper

Plant: Black Pepper

Botanical name: Piper nigrum

Origins: Distilled from the dried black pepper berries (peppercorns).

Aroma: Hot and spicy.

Properties: Appetite stimulant, antiseptic and digestive.

Uses: Excellent for muscular aches and rheumatism, loss of appetite and chilblains.

Suggested Blends: Frankincense, sandalwood, lavender and rosemary.

Perfume Note: Middle

Plant: Citronella

Botanical name: Cymbopogon nardus

Origins: Extracted from the top of the grass.

Aroma: Sharp and lemony.

Properties: Insect repelling and a tonic.

Uses: An excellent scent for your garden candles guaranteed to keep those summer barbecue bugs at bay.

Suggested Blends:
Lavender and rosemary.

Perfume Note: Top

WARNING!
Do NOT use if you are pregnant.

Plant: Clove

Botanical name: Eugenia caryophyllata

Origins: Extracted from the flower buds of the clove tree.

Aroma: Slightly bitter and woody.

WARNING!
Do NOT apply directly to skin or inhale via steam applications – best to use as a room scent or fumigant only.

Properties: Antiseptic and anti-rheumatic.

Uses: A classic remedy for toothache, neuralgia, arthritis and rheumatism. Repels clothes moths.

Suggested Blends: Orange, rose otto and ylang ylang.

Perfume Note: Middle

Plant: Fennel

Botanical name: Foeniculum vulgare

Origins: Distilled from the crushed seeds.

Aroma: Aniseed

Properties: Anti-inflammatory and a tonic.

Uses: This is used as a tonic for the digestive system and to treat premenstrual problems.

Suggested Blends:
Lavender, geranium and rose otto

Perfume Note: Top/middle

WARNING!
Do NOT use if you are either pregnant or epileptic.

Plant: Ginger

Botanical name: Zingiber officinalis

Origins: Distilled from the dried rhizomes of the plant.

Aroma: Earthy and spicy.

Properties: Antiseptic and stimulant.

Uses: A wonderful remedy for nausea and for catarrh, congestion and coughs.

Suggested Blends: Grapefruit, geranium, spearmint and patchouli

Perfume Note: Middle/base

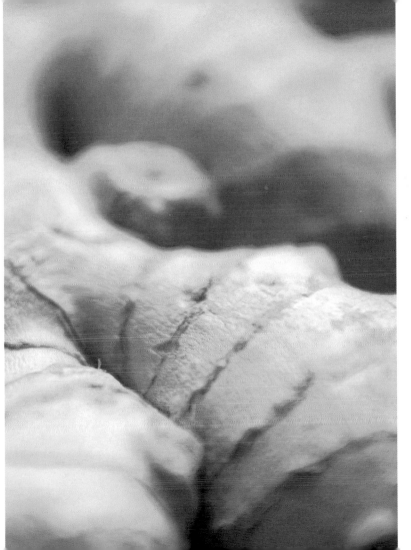

> **WARNING!**
> Do NOT use
> if you are
> pregnant.

Plant: Jasmine

Botanical name: Jasminum officinalis

Origins: Extracted from flowers picked after dusk when the oil is at its highest concentration.

Aroma: Heady, exotic and floral.

Properties: Sedative and antidepressant.

Uses: An excellent tonic for premenstrual syndrome and depression.

Suggested Blends: Camomile, ylang ylang and sandalwood.

Perfume Note: Middle

Plant: Juniper

Botanical name: Juniperus communis

Origins: Extracted from the crushed or dried berries.

Aroma: Fresh and woody.

Properties: Antiseptic and sedative.

Uses: This is beneficial in treating skin, arthritis and rheumatic conditions.

Suggested Blends: Rose otto, clary sage, geranium, grapefruit and lemon.

Perfume Note: Middle

WARNING!
Do NOT use if you are pregnant.

Plant: Lemon grass

Botanical name: Cymbopogon citratus

Origins: Extracted from the oriental grass.

Aroma: Sweet and lemony.

Properties: Insecticidal, antiseptic and a tonic.

Uses: This is good for relieving stress and palpitations. It will also stimulate breast milk in nursing mothers.

Suggested Blends: Geranium, myrrh, palmarosa and petitgrain.

Perfume Note: Top

Plant: Marjoram

Botanical name: Origanum marjorana

Origins: Extracted from the leaves.

Aroma: Herbaceous, warm and spicy.

Properties: Digestive, antiseptic and sedative.

Uses: It lowers blood pressure, eases muscle injuries and sprains and aids insomnia.

Suggested Blends: Juniper, tea tree and rosemary.

Perfume Note: Middle

107

Plant: Myrrh

Botanical name: Commiphora myrrha

Origins: Extracted from the gum resin of the bark stem.

Aroma: Smoky and balsamic.

Properties: Anti-inflammatory, antiseptic and sedative.

Uses: This is excellent for healing wounds and in caring for cracked skin and scars.

Suggested Blends: Cedarwood, frankincense, lemon grass and patchouli.

Perfume Note: Base

Plant: Niaouli

Botanical name: Melaleuca viridiflora

Origins: Extracted from the young twigs and leaves of the tree.

Aroma: Strong and camphoraceous.

Properties: Antiseptic and digestive.

Uses: For bronchial conditions and insect bites. This is a common ingredient in mouthwashes and toothpastes and has been used to purify water.

Suggested Blends: Peppermint, juniper and lavender.

Perfume Note: Middle

Plant: Palmarosa

Botanical name: Cymbopogon martini

Origins: Extracted from the fragrant grass, related to citronella and lemon grass.

Aroma: Geranium-like and sweet.

Properties: Antidepressant and a tonic.

Uses: Will aid nervous exhaustion and stress, and is also used to treat oily skin, acne and dermatitis.

Suggested Blends: Cedarwood, lavender and ylang ylang.

Perfume Note: Middle

Plant: Patchouli

Botanical name: Pogostemon cablin

Origins: Distilled from the soft furry leaves which evoke the fragrance when rubbed.

Aroma: Earthy, musky and improves with age.

Properties: Stimulant, antidepressant and a tonic.

Uses: Used to treat dermatitis, abscesses, athlete's foot, nausea, and travel sickness.

Suggested Blends: Geranium, cedarwood and tea tree.

Perfume Note: Base

Plant: Petitgrain

Botanical name: Citrus aurantium

Origins: Extracted from the leaves and twigs of the same tree which produces neroli oil.

Aroma: Bittersweet

Properties: Digestive and antiseptic.

Uses: This makes an excellent antidepressant, and is recommended for treating acne.

Suggested Blends: Clary sage, geranium, lavender and rosemary.

Perfume Note: Top

115

WARNING!
Do NOT use if you are pregnant.

Plant: Rosewood

Botanical name: Aniba rosaeodora

Origins: Extracted from the chipping of the rosewood tree.

Aroma: Soft and woody.

Properties: Boosts the immune system and makes a good antidepressant.

Uses: Use this to rejuvenate mature skin. It also helps to prevent colds and flu.

Suggested Blends: Lavender, jasmine, tangerine, grapefruit and lemon.

Perfume Note: Middle

117

Plant: Spearmint

Botanical name: Mentha spicata

Origins: Steam distilled from the flower tops.

Aroma: Warm, herbaceous and mint-scented.

Properties: Digestive and a tonic.

Uses: A good treatment for headaches and nausea, and it is used in the treatment of dermatitis.

Suggested Blends: Tea tree, lavender, rosemary and geranium.

Perfume Note: Top

Plant: Tangerine

Botanical name: Citrus reticulata

Origins: Extracted from the peel of the fruit.

Aroma: Fruity and sweet.

Properties: Digestive

Uses: This is good for helping circulation, combating constipation and diarrhoea. It is also used to keep stretch marks at bay.

Suggested Blends: Orange and neroli.

Perfume Note: Top

122

Plant: Thyme

Botanical name: Thymus vulgaris

Origins: Steam distilled from fresh or partly dried leaves and flower tops.

Aroma: Spicy and herbaceous.

Properties: Antiseptic, diuretic, anti-rheumatic and fungicidal.

Uses: Recommended for respiratory problems including bronchitis and asthma.

Suggested Blends: Lemon, marjoram, rosemary and lavender.

Perfume Note: Middle

Plant: Vetiver

Botanical name: Vetiveria zizanioides

Origins: Related to palmarosa and lemon grass, vetiver is extracted from the dried and chopped (highly fragrant) roots of the grass plant

Aroma: Earthy and rich – improving with age.

Properties: The 'oil of tranquillity' is renowned for its calming effect and is a reputed aphrodisiac!

Uses: A popular fixative in the perfume industry.

Suggested Blends: Sandalwood, lavender and ylang ylang.

Perfume Note: Base

125

✓ Always do a patch test before using any essential oil (see page 11).

✓ Always dilute in a carrier oil before applying to your skin.

✓ Always keep essential oil away from your eyes and do not rub your eyes after handling them.

✓ If you are pregnant seek medical advice before using essential oils.

✓ If you are epileptic seek medical advice before using essential oils.

✗ Never take essential oils by mouth, rectum or vagina unless medically instructed to do so.

✗ Never use citrus oils on the skin shortly before exposure to the sun. Citrus oils increase skin sensitivity to the sun and use may cause pigmentation.

✗ Avoid citrus oils if you have a history of melanoma.

✗ Never use an essential oil if you can find little information about it.

✗ Avoid prolonged use of the same essential oil.

✗ If you are asthmatic avoid steam inhalations.

Care for your essential oils and they will care for you!

- ✿ Essential oils are light sensitive so store them in dark glass bottles with stoppers.
- ✿ Store in a cool, dark place.
- ✿ Keep out of reach of children.
- ✿ Do not keep oils in the bathroom where they will evaporate and become stale from the steam.
- ✿ Essential oils can last for up to 2 years if kept chilled.
- ✿ If you wish to keep them in the refrigerator, take them out an hour or so before using so that they will flow freely.
- ✿ Some essential oils improve with age – sandalwood, patchouli, and frankincense for instance.
- ✿ Essential oils in the citrus family last no longer than six months.